AF484181

TO:23

Health Coach Guide Weight Management

United Health Coach

Copyright © 2018 United Health Coach

All rights reserved.

CHAPTER THREE: LOSING WEIGHT

Losing weight is not only a matter of diet and exercise. There are countless things around and in between needed to achieve a healthy weight. As this program suggests, it's about: *social skills, dietary education, stress control, having the right tools and more.* Having a grasp on what details weight loss, will help you set realistic and healthy goals.

For most of us in this program, losing weight is the goal. Although losing weight can be a solution to many things, it's important to know that not all weight loss is created equal. This chapter will discuss what losing weight means, the basic science to achieve it, and how to support it.

Here you will learn:

- What is a safe amount of weight to lose?

- The math and science behind weight loss

- Some of the many benefits to losing weight

- The difference between weight loss and being healthy

- How diet and exercise impacts weight loss

~ ~ ~

Losing weight is easy. The problem is, it's easier not too

– Inspired by Jim Rohn

~ ~ ~

WEIGHT LOSS: THE VAGUE STATEMENT

Most often when someone says they want to lose weight, what they really mean is a desire to lose fat. To "lose weight" is a vague statement and sometimes can lead to unhealthy decisions to lose fat. One of the more common examples can be seen in people who promote sweating in attempt to shed fat pounds. Excessive sweating from saunas, plastic clothing and such, may help you temporarily lose weight, and perhaps inches but you will not lose fat.

Sweating and fat loss are associated, but sweating does not cause fat loss: causality. The act of sweating is a reaction from the body in an attempt to cool down when a body reaches a certain temperature. A raised temperature can be caused by many different factors such as: fighting infection, an external heat source, or activity. Although all of these things can cause you to lose weight, only one will trigger fat stores to convert to more energy (fat loss).

Being specific and using a well-guided diet and exercise program will ensure the best results. It is important to identify your <u>true</u> goals and intentions and use that to measure your success. If your goal is to lose inches around your waist, then measure your waist and go from there. Similarly, if the goal is blood pressure or blood sugar improvement, measure those things and look for change in these areas.

Beyond the math and vague expression, weight loss can be simple. How or how much you lose can be the more complex part. How you go about losing weight will determine several things such as: health risks, level of satisfaction and longevity.

Research proves that losing weight too quickly most often results in regain of weight (rebound). At very best, rapid weight loss makes it that much more difficult to maintain. The reason behind this fact is that rapid weight loss creates a shock to the body, and it will respond by attempting to stay at status quo.

Imagine having a savings account that has been suddenly depleted. The natural response is to panic and make every attempt to hold on to your money. This is the shock response. Using the same analogy, you will see that if money was withdrawn in small frequent amounts, it would be easy to go unnoticed.

Shock from rapid weight loss not only may sabotage your maintenance, it can also create unhealthy conditions and disease. In short, it is unhealthy. This is why research proves that slow and steady weight loss is not only healthier but will promote sustainable weight loss.

DAILY INTAKE

Your daily recommended calorie intake is the amount of calories you need for an average day. Eating more than your recommended amount will result in weight gain, while eating less will result in weight loss. Although this formula is dynamic and can vary, it's important to have an idea of what your estimated calorie need will be.

The amount of calories a person needs will always vary depending on weight, height, muscle to fat ratio and level of activity. To find out you recommended daily calorie intake simply go online and search for: "calorie intake calculator".

The goal is to maintain an intake amount equal to or less than your daily recommended amount. In order to so, you will first need pertinent information such as calorie amount in each food versus your recommended amount.

Calorie intake calculators use the same formula so you should find the same results regardless of the source. Just be sure not to apply to a service or provide more than the anonymous information needed.

What is your daily need?

DOING THE MATH: WEIGHT LOSS

Understanding weight loss on a mathematical level is non-complex. It is basic subtraction. Eat fewer calories than needed or burn more than you take in and you will lose weight. This is simple math at its finest.

Let's take a look at an equation that you should familiarize yourself with. This is the equation for the metric value of one pound (2.2 kg). One pound is roughly equal to **3500 calories.** This means that a person would need to deplete 3500 calories in order to lose one pound or eat in excess to gain one pound. (Be mindful that this is mostly achieved over the course of days or weeks).

A person could lose weight by either forgoing an additional 3500 calories or burning an additional 3500. Although either of the two methods work well individually, the most effective way to lose weight is in the combination of both. That is, take in slightly less calories than needed while at the same time burning slightly more that you take in.

The standard recommendation for a safe weight loss is usually a combined calorie deficit of **250 calories** per day and an additional burning of **250 calories**, equaling a total of **500 calories a day**. This would result in a minimum one-pound loss per week (500 x 7 days = 3500).

It's good to note that 250 calories in either direction is small but can add up to a big difference. Later you will learn effective ways to avoid a minimum of 250 calories daily and also how to burn 250 calories with little effort. For example: an hour of brisk walking and eliminating one can of soda will equal 500 calorie daily deficit!

WEIGHT LOSS BENEFITS

Short of being a sumo wrestler, there are very few benefits to being overweight. On the contrary there are many health risks associated. Being overweight or obese can decrease your quality of life through weight related complications. Excess weight-bearing can cause discomfort and also decrease physical performance.

Health risks include but not limited to: diabetes, high blood pressure, depression, heart disease and premature death. Apart from physical health risks, being at an unhealthy weight can lead to social and financial issues such as isolation and increased medical cost.

There are countless reasons to be at a healthy weight. Within limited exception, there is very little that healthy weight loss won't fix or make better. The benefits are endless. You will encounter many reasons that may motivate you but remember that the most important reasons are the ones that are specific to you.

The number of benefits can be endless. Increased energy, improved appearance, increased self-esteem are just to name a few. It's also worth noting that one benefit typically leads to another, which in turn leads to another benefit, and so on. This is called a ***positive cycle*** of health.

POSITIVE AND NEGATIVE CYCLE

Of the many benefits of losing weight, the cumulative effects of all, heavily outweigh any one specific benefit. There are many lanes of health such as: mental, physical and financial health, yet it's important to understand that they all interchangeably affect each other. How you look affects how you feel, and how you feel can affect your level of financial success and so forth. Ultimately this course empowers and repeats. This is called a cycle.

A cycle, like any wheel, has the ability to spin in either direction, for good or bad. Because it is a continuous loop, the cycle can begin at any point within its circle. The reverse is true as well as a cycle can be broken at any point.

Let's look at an example of both a negative and positive cycle.

NEGATIVE CYCLE EXAMPLE

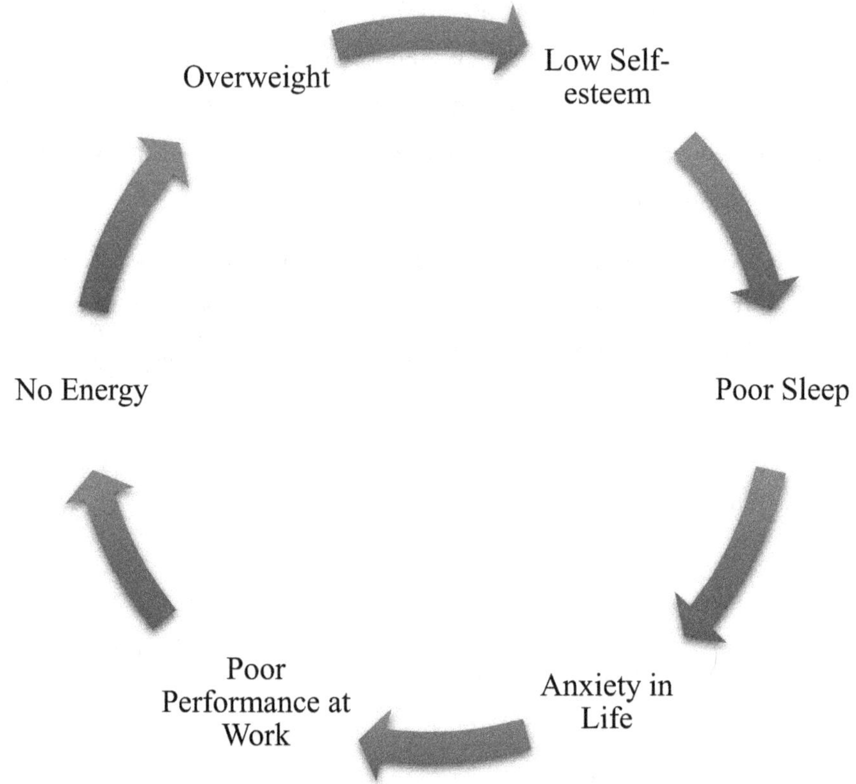

For this example:

- A person who is overweight will likely have low energy

- Low/no energy can lead to poor performance at work

- Poor work performance can lead to work stress and anxiety

- Stress and anxiety can lead to sleep issues (over or under sleeping)

- Poor sleep habits can affect mood and confidence

- Lack of confidence and motivation… the cycle continues...

POSITIVE CYCLE EXAMPLE

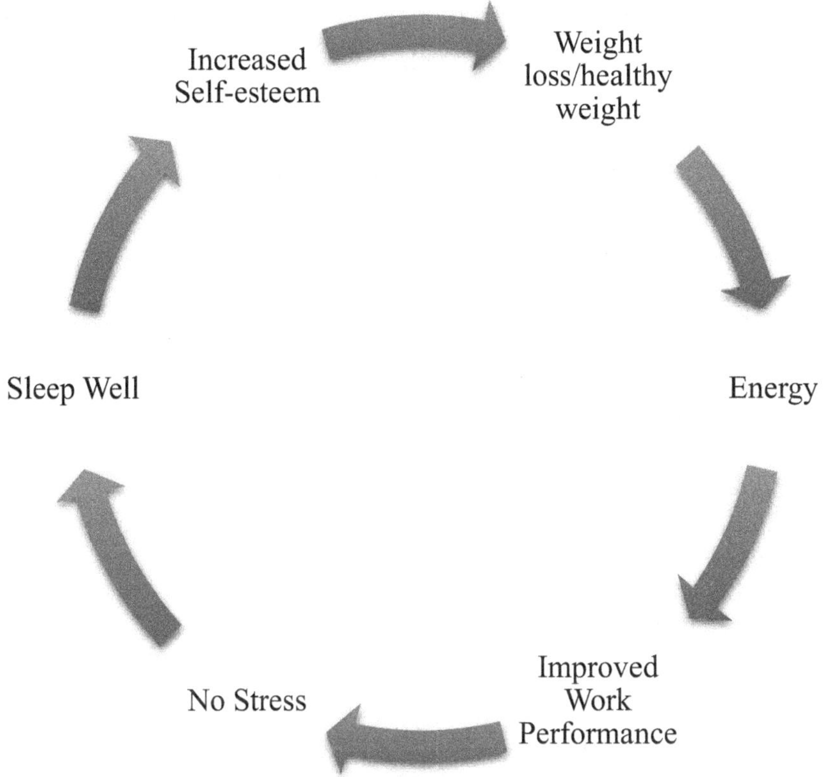

For this example:

- Losing weight increases energy

- Increased energy yields better work performance and attitude

- Better work performance leads to less stress

- Lack of stress helps you sleep well

- Good sleep hygiene supports mood and self-esteem

- High self-esteem and energy lead to success…

WHAT DOES BEING HEALTHY MEAN?

A healthy life reaches beyond a weight but yet for many of us, being healthy means being thin. Although it's true that being overweight can increase your chances of developing health risks but being thin alone doesn't ensure you will be healthy.

Being healthy means having healthy habits. Living a lifestyle that is conducive to your well-being. It is not limited to the hour or so spent during a healthy activity, but rather how you spend your entire day, every day.

There are many things that encompass a healthy lifestyle such as:

- Not smoking

- Healthy diet (next chapter)

- Limiting alcohol consumption

- Daily exercise or activity

- Stress management

Quality of life should be your main focus in maintaining health. No matter your reasons for making change, ultimately its purpose is to serve as a medium of satisfaction. That is to say, lower blood pressure, sugar, waistline or pounds in the end will make you happy. Being happy is being healthy.

WHAT IS A HEALTHY WEIGHT?

A healthy weight is a range that puts your body in an optimal environment to thrive and endure fewer complications. We know that too much fat is not healthy and can cause complications, as well as not enough fat can also have health risks. So, the question remains, what is a healthy weight?

As you learned earlier, medical science states that a healthy weight is a BMI target range of **18.5 - 25** and a body fat percentage of around **10 - 22%** for men and slightly more for women (depending on age). Although the standard BMI measurement is not perfect, it does provide a good guideline for recognizing weight associated health risks, being that people who register out of range have been shown to have increased health risks.

While weight plays a significant role in our health, the greatest health risks are related to: smoking, diet, and inactivity. Whether you are over, under or at a healthy weight, you are still at increased risk of complications or premature death by having an unhealthy diet, smoking cigarettes and having a sedentary lifestyle.

No matter what weight you carry, you will always be healthier by living a healthy lifestyle that includes a healthy diet, daily activity and <u>NOT</u> smoking! If you are considered overweight but follow a healthy lifestyle, chances are you will be healthier than someone who is at a normal weight but has poor habits.

Genetics also play a role in our health. It is said that 70% of weight is hereditary. Therefore, the genes we inherit can override many health choices we make. This is why it's important to tell your healthcare provider all the details of your family health history. Along with a healthy lifestyle, your provider may prescribe medication that will improve your health or prevent certain complications.

Understanding that a healthy weight for one person may not be healthy for another. Sometimes accepting that you may not be as thin as you'd envision may be healthier than forcing an unnatural weight loss. If your body is in optimal health and you are not at risk of developing health conditions, looking for more weight loss can be counterproductive or dangerous. Your perception of healthy weight may be unhealthy or not realistic; therefor, always work with your healthcare provider or professional to coach you.

How you look and feel is perhaps more important than what you weigh. Weight is not only subjective but also insufficient information in determining health. As long as you are doing all the things in life that are healthy, your weight may be of less concern.

Again, healthy habits include: stress management, healthy eating, daily activity, limiting alcohol and not smoking. Doing these things will not guarantee "perfect" health (as nothing will), but it will guarantee you will be at _your_ best health.

~ ~ ~

Aim to be healthy... Weight loss is merely a by-product

- Healthy Fact!

~ ~ ~

TO23 ACTIVITIES WEEK THREE

ACTIVITY ONE: CHECK-IN

1. Where you successful in your action plan? (Answer one)

   a. Yes! Congratulations!

   b. Not successful. Unfortunate, but with every failure is an opportunity to learn

2. What were the barriers?

Can you *problem-solve*? If yes, problem solve below.

Possible Solutions	**Confidence Score**

Choose one:

Will you try it? | YES | NO

Is your solution **SMART?** | YES | NO

What did you learn?

ACTIVITY TWO: ACTION PLAN

Suggested Action Plan, Meal Prep: Snack is a word that should be redefined. What some consider as snacks in most cases are usually high caloric, low nutritional value foods. Remember that the purpose of eating is to supply energy and building material for your body.

Most snacks that we eat are sufficient enough to be considered a meal. The problem with considering a meal a snack is that it sends a message to the brain that calorie intake may have been insufficient, creating a desire to eat more. Redefining your definition of what a snack is means understanding that you have a large enough of calorie intake to suffice until next meal.

Example: ***Eating an apple***

Referring to an apple as a snack between breakfast and lunch leaves you feeling as though you had insufficient food, therefore you may have a larger lunch. Whereas, considering it a 2nd meal will leave you feeling content and will not impact your lunch decision. Know that an apple has sufficient calorie and carbohydrate value to sustain you through to your next meal.

Small nutrient dense meals should be eaten every 3- 4 hours. As you learn next chapter (NUTRITION), larger meals should be eaten earlier in the day and tapered down towards the evening where less energy is needed.

Avoid grazing between meals. Rather save all calorie intake for meals at designated times. One way to ensure you are consuming the right foods is to prepare meals in advance. Your suggested action plan for this week is to work on meal prep.

You can choose this suggested action plan or create an entirely new action plan. The choice is yours. Just know that the goal is to move forward towards greater health. **Good luck!**

Using the SMART criteria, make an Action plan for the week

What will you do?

How long you will do it for?

How many times per week?

Your confidence level 0-10? _________

If your confidence level is below seven, considering modifying the action plan until your confidence level is at a seven or greater.

Example:

I will ride my bike for 30 minutes per day, 3 days out of the week. My confidence in completing this action plan is 9 out of 10!

Be Ultimate! – Be You

ACTIVITY THREE: BEING HEALTHY [WRITING ASSIGNMENT]

Before you get healthy you must first know what healthy looks like. Below, in your own words describe what healthy means to you.

How will you know when you are healthy?

What does healthy look like on you?

ACTIVITY FOUR: FOOD LOG

Let's gather some vital information on the food you eat. If a better diet is needed, it's important to know where the corrections can be made. Remembering that nutrition will dictate your overall health. Understanding what is in your food will help you create better strategies to health implementation.

Keep a food log for five days (minimum 3 days). Chart down everything that goes into your mouth. Include the following information: fat, protein, carbohydrate and calories. You can web search your food item, or use easy-to-use apps such as Myfitnesspal to track everything for you. Either way, it will get easier to track each additional day.

Next chapter you will learn details in your choices and how to make better choices if needed.

Breakfast	Fat (grams)	Protein (grams)	Carbohydrates	Calories
Snack	Fat (grams)	Protein (grams)	Carbohydrates	Calories
Lunch	Fat (grams)	Protein (grams)	Carbohydrates	Calories
Snack	Fat (grams)	Protein (grams)	Carbohydrates	Calories
Dinner	Fat (grams)	Protein (grams)	Carbohydrates	Calories
Other	Fat (grams)	Protein (grams)	Carbohydrates	Calories
Total				

Breakfast	Fat (grams)	Protein (grams)	Carbohydrates	Calories
Snack	Fat (grams)	Protein (grams)	Carbohydrates	Calories
Lunch	Fat (grams)	Protein (grams)	Carbohydrates	Calories
Snack	Fat (grams)	Protein (grams)	Carbohydrates	Calories
Dinner	Fat (grams)	Protein (grams)	Carbohydrates	Calories
Other	Fat (grams)	Protein (grams)	Carbohydrates	Calories
Total				

Breakfast	Fat (grams)	Protein (grams)	Carbohydrates	Calories
Snack	Fat (grams)	Protein (grams)	Carbohydrates	Calories
Lunch	Fat (grams)	Protein (grams)	Carbohydrates	Calories
Snack	Fat (grams)	Protein (grams)	Carbohydrates	Calories
Dinner	Fat (grams)	Protein (grams)	Carbohydrates	Calories
Other	Fat (grams)	Protein (grams)	Carbohydrates	Calories
Total				

Breakfast	Fat (grams)	Protein (grams)	Carbohydrates	Calories

Snack	Fat (grams)	Protein (grams)	Carbohydrates	Calories

Lunch	Fat (grams)	Protein (grams)	Carbohydrates	Calories

Snack	Fat (grams)	Protein (grams)	Carbohydrates	Calories

Dinner	Fat (grams)	Protein (grams)	Carbohydrates	Calories

Other	Fat (grams)	Protein (grams)	Carbohydrates	Calories
Total				

Breakfast	Fat (grams)	Protein (grams)	Carbohydrates	Calories
Snack	Fat (grams)	Protein (grams)	Carbohydrates	Calories
Lunch	Fat (grams)	Protein (grams)	Carbohydrates	Calories
Snack	Fat (grams)	Protein (grams)	Carbohydrates	Calories
Dinner	Fat (grams)	Protein (grams)	Carbohydrates	Calories
Other	Fat (grams)	Protein (grams)	Carbohydrates	Calories
Total				

ACTION PLAN SUGGESTIONS

- Because calories are intended to fuel our activities, we require less towards the end of the day. Consider an action plan that involves not eating late nights (2-4 hours prior to sleep).

- Add calorie-burning exercises as a nearly daily routine. The national recommendation suggests 150 minutes per week. The most standard version of this is 5 days of 30 minutes of moderate exercise per week.

- You can find all the nutrients you need in a delicious smoothie for less calories and fat. Replace one meal a day for a healthy fruit and vegetable smoothie. Add protein for muscle sustenance.

- Switch out sugary beverages (iced tea, soda, fruit juices etc.) for water, flavored water or other no calorie drink.

- Replace one meal a day for a healthy all-green plate. The word salad can sound boring to some. Choose an array of vegetables to spice it up.

- Reduce or eliminate refined foods. Especially sugary snacks (donuts, cookies, crackers, white breads etc.) as a plan.

- Portion control without measuring. Simply make or order your typical meal, but only eat 50-75%. Wrap the rest up for later.

- Get more sleep. You burn calories more efficiently while sleeping. Also, because you are sleeping you are not eating.

- Increase your water intake. Water helps keep you satiated and is calorie free. Also has endless other benefits!

- Add strength-training exercises. Larger muscles burn more calories during and post exercise.

- If you are a drinker know that alcohol has multiple weight-loss prohibiting effects. Reducing or eliminating alcohol is a great way to lose weight. Make alcohol management a plan.

~ ~ ~

Always plan ahead. It wasn't raining when Noah built the ark!

- Richard Cushing

~ ~ ~

www.ingramcontent.com/pod-product-compliance
Lightning Source LLC
Chambersburg PA
CBHW071506150726
48000CB00006B/2725